TEN RULES FOR GUARANTEED WEIGHT LOSS

BULLET GUIDE

Hodder Education, 338 Euston Road, London NW1 3BH

Hodder Education is an Hachette UK company

First published in UK 2011 by Hodder Education

This edition published 2011

Copyright © 2011 Sara Kirkham

The moral rights of the author have been asserted.

Database right Hodder Education (makers)

Artworks (internal and cover): Peter Lubach
Cover concept design: Two Associates

All rights reserved. No part of this publication may be reproduced, stored in a retrieval system or transmitted in any form or by any means, electronic, mechanical, photocopying, recording or otherwise, without the prior permission in writing of Hodder Education, or as expressly permitted by law, or under terms agreed with the appropriate reprographic rights organization. Enquiries concerning reproduction outside the scope of the above should be sent to the Rights Department, Hodder Education, at the address above.

You must not circulate this book in any other binding or cover and you must impose this same condition on any acquirer.

British Library Cataloguing in Publication Data: a catalogue record for this title is available from the British Library.

10 9 8 7 6 5 4 3 2 1

The publisher has used its best endeavours to ensure that any website addresses referred to in this book are correct and active at the time of going to press. However, the publisher and the author have no responsibility for the websites and can make no guarantee that a site will remain live or that the content will remain relevant, decent or appropriate.

The publisher has made every effort to mark as such all words which it believes to be trademarks. The publisher should also like to make it clear that the presence of a word in the book, whether marked or unmarked, in no way affects its legal status as a trademark.

Every reasonable effort has been made by the publisher to trace the copyright holders of material in this book. Any errors or omissions should be notified in writing to the publisher, who will endeavour to rectify the situation for any reprints and future editions.

Hachette UK's policy is to use papers that are natural, renewable and recyclable products and made from wood grown in sustainable forests. The logging and manufacturing processes are expected to conform to the environmental regulations of the country of origin.

www.hoddereducation.co.uk

Typeset by Stephen Rowling/Springworks

Printed in Spain

TEN RULES FOR GUARANTEED WEIGHT LOSS

BULLET GUIDE

Sara Kirkham

About the author

Sara Kirkham is a nutritionist, writer and lecturer with over 20 years' experience of helping people to lose weight. Sara has written and delivered nutrition modules for colleges and universities, has published several books on weight loss and nutrition, and writes nutrition articles for newspapers and websites. She has a First-class Honours degree in Nutritional Medicine, and has had research published in the *Journal of Diabetes, Obesity and Metabolism*.

As well as helping clients to lose weight in her nutritional practice, she also runs regular weight loss courses online and in her local area, and delivers weight loss workshops at boot camps. With a background in exercise instruction and years of experience in helping people to adapt their diet and exercise lifestyle, Sara aims to capture all that practical information, expertise and experience in *Ten Rules for Guaranteed Weight Loss*, providing you with a quick and effective guide to losing weight.

Contents

1 Balancing calories — 1
2 Measuring weight loss — 13
3 Setting a weight loss goal — 25
4 Fail to plan, plan to fail — 37
5 Reducing calorie intake — 49
6 Portion control — 61
7 Increasing calorie expenditure — 73
8 Manipulating protein and carbohydrate intake for results — 85
9 Jumping over hurdles for long-term success — 97
10 A diet for life — 109

Introduction

In a world saturated with dietary advice, *Ten Rules for Guaranteed Weight Loss* provides you with the quickest, healthiest and most effective way of losing weight and keeping it off for life. It offers a credible source of information with a wealth of practical tips, giving you all the tools you need for successful weight loss.

Almost 50% of women are dieting most of the time, with 13 million people in the UK on a permanent diet, and yet more people than ever are overweight. Diet plans promising radical weight loss are too good to be true. This book is for you if you want to lose weight and maintain a healthy weight for life.

If you consume fewer calories than you use up, you lose weight, but we often set ambitious weight loss goals, follow diets that cannot be sustained, and begin vigorous exercise regimes that were never going to last more than a week. Changing eating and exercise habits and adapting food choices is tough, but follow the ten golden rules for weight loss in this guide, and you will lose weight:

* Reduce calories without being 'on a diet'.
* Find out what you need to lose.
* Set weight loss goals to help you succeed.
* Get organized.
* Balance calorie intake and expenditure without reducing metabolism.
* Adapt *how* you eat, not just *what* you eat, for portion control.
* Begin and stick with an effective weight loss exercise regime.
* Learn how to get over diet hurdles that interfere with success.
* Make small, achievable changes that become habitual, then make more changes on top of these.
* Discover the weight loss benefits of higher protein diets without the health risks – follow a healthy diet that *can* be sustained.

This *Bullet Guide* is guaranteed to give you weight loss success if you follow it!

1 Balancing calories

The biggest question on everyone's lips is how to lose weight and keep it off – the solution is simple, but not necessarily easy! However, with a little know-how you can **balance calorie intake and expenditure**, lose weight, and keep it off for life.

There are three reasons for weight gain:

1 eating high-calorie foods
2 large portion sizes
3 not being active enough.

The energy balance equation states: if calorie intake is less than calorie expenditure, you will lose weight

Most people try to **reduce calorie intake** in order to lose weight – a good idea if you are consuming too many calories to begin with.

> **Calorie counts**
> Fats   9 calories per gram
> Carbohydrates   4 calories per gram
> Protein   4 calories per gram
> Alcohol   7 calories per gram

A **calorie** is the amount of energy required to raise the temperature of 1 gram of water by 1°C. It is our body's energy currency – we take food in, digest and store it, and use it for energy. The kilojoule is another metric measurement of food energy – one kilocalorie (dietary calorie) is equivalent to approximately 4.2 kilojoules.

Weight control is about balancing your **calorie intake** against your **calorie expenditure**. This is known as the **energy balance equation**.

If calories in equal calories out, your weight remains the same.
If calorie intake exceeds calorie expenditure, you gain weight.
If calorie intake is less than calorie expenditure, you lose weight.

So this means that, to lose weight, you have to:

* reduce calorie intake *or*
* increase calorie expenditure *or*
* do both.

It sounds simple, doesn't it?

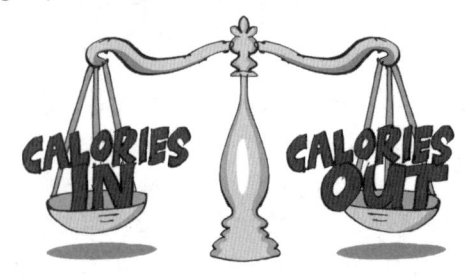

Many things affect **food choices** and **exercise**, and we often think we have eaten less and exercised more. Take a look at these common **weight loss pitfalls** …

- **restrictive diet plans** that cannot be maintained, leading to **gorging on foods** you are craving
- following **low-calorie diets that reduce blood sugar levels**, causing higher food intake at the next meal
- **not counting** the odd glass of wine, chips off someone else's plate, a handful of crisps …
- **convincing yourself** that you'll go to the gym tomorrow instead – which never happens!

Although the **energy balance equation** is simple and effective, creating a **calorie deficit** can be challenging.

Your **basal metabolic rate (BMR)** is the number of calories needed daily at rest, taking account of age, weight and gender.

Females

Age	Basal metabolic rate
10–17	Weight in kg multiplied by 13.4 + 692
18–29	Weight in kg multiplied by 14.8 + 487
30–59	Weight in kg multiplied by 8.3 + 846
60–74	Weight in kg multiplied by 9.2 + 687
75+	Weight in kg multiplied by 9.8 + 624

Males

Age	Basal metabolic rate
10–17	Weight in kg multiplied by 17.7 + 657
18–29	Weight in kg multiplied by 15.1 + 692
30–59	Weight in kg multiplied by 11.5 + 873
60–74	Weight in kg multiplied by 11.9 + 700
75+	Weight in kg multiplied by 8.4 + 821

Source: Modified Schofield equations. Department of Health (1991).
© Crown copyright. Licensed under the Open Government Licence v.1.0

A common error is to **reduce calorie intake too low** in order to lose weight more quickly. If calorie intake is reduced to less than the amount of energy your body needs to function at rest (your **BMR**) for too long, your body will begin to **use less energy** and **store more fat**.

In this situation, you use muscle for energy, which **decreases metabolic rate** and the number of calories used over a 24 hour period – bad news if you want to lose weight, as you want your **metabolic rate** to be higher, not lower.

Remember that your BMR is the number of calories you need at your current weight for weight maintenance. As you lose weight, your caloric requirements also reduce

Adapting calorie intake for weight loss

With **regular exercise** your calorie requirement is higher, but to **lose weight** you need to **consume fewer calories than you expend**. Consuming the exact number of calories you need (with or without exercise) will **maintain** your current weight. You need to **take in fewer calories, or use up more,** to reduce body weight.

Remember – your **BMR** is based on current body weight: as you **lose weight you require fewer calories** (a lighter body is easier to move around). This is one reason why **weight loss will plateau** if calorie intake is not adjusted as weight is lost. However, you cannot keep reducing calorie intake, and this is where **regular exercise** comes in.

Bullet Guide: Ten Rules for Guaranteed Weight Loss

Counting calories

The benefit of **calorie counting** is that, if you get it right, you should be able to control your weight. However, counting calories can be hard work.

You need to:

1 Calculate an accurate **BMR**.
2 **Weigh foods** for accurate calorie counts.
3 Choose the correct food **brands** if using books or websites to calculate calorie intake.
4 **Be 100% honest** and include everything you have eaten and drunk.

Although it can be time consuming, you will learn the calorie content of foods and drinks, and can adapt your diet accordingly. However, not all low-calorie, diet foods are good for you, and not all high-calorie foods are bad for you (e.g. fish, avocados, nuts).

Food marketing can be deceptive – **low-calorie/-fat** foods might not be all that they seem. **'Reduced calorie'** foods should contain **25% fewer calories** than the standard version, but the **serving size** is often very small. If you eat more, you will not benefit from the low calorie intake.

TOP TIP

Compare **calories per serving** between products – some 'diet' foods are:

* barely **lower in fat and/or calories** than other products
* lower in fat, but **added sugar** stops them being low calorie
* lower in calories/fat than a **standard version** of the same food, but if the **standard version is high in calories/fat**, the 'diet' version may not be that great!

'Light' or 'lite' products must have at least **30% less** fat, sugar or calories than standard products.

High-fat products such as mayonnaise may be labelled 'reduced fat/calorie' but are still a high-fat food if the fat content exceeds 20 grams fat per 100 grams.

High-fat products contain more than 20 g fat per 100 g. Low-fat products contain 3 g or less fat per 100 g.

Nutrient content	Calories/100g	Fat content (g/100 g)	Sugar content (g/100 g)	Sodium (g/100 g)
Normal mayonnaise	724	79.3	0.1	0.24
Low-fat mayonnaise	288	28.1	4.6	0.94

If you are relying on food labelling to provide you with accurate information, you have to learn to read between the lines!

2 Measuring weight loss

There are several ways to **measure** weight loss progress; although you don't have to weigh or measure yourself, it's good to have a **starting point** and a **goal** so you know that you are heading in the right direction.

Body measurement options include:

1. weighing scales
2. body mass index
3. tape measurements
4. body fat measurements.

It's not how heavy you are that matters, it's how much of you is fat

There are benefits and drawbacks to all types of measurement, but each provides a **starting point** and has **'norm' values**, which you should aim to reach to achieve better health.

Benefits and drawbacks of measuring instruments

Type of measurement	✓	✗
Tape measurements	Quick and easy	Can be inaccurate
Scales	Quick and easy Should be accurate	Measure overall body weight rather than fat loss
Body mass index (BMI)	Easy with charts or on-line calculators	Only based upon weight and height
Body fat measurements	Specifically measures body fat	Accuracy is affected by body hydration levels

Weighing scales

Weighing scales are the most popular way of measuring weight loss, although you are weighing muscle, bone mass, water and fat, so the proportion of body fat remains unknown.

Tips for accurate weighing

* Make sure the **pointer** is set to zero on non-electronic scales.
* If the reading on electronic scales fluctuates or seems inaccurate, **check the battery.**
* **Stand upright** – leaning forwards or backwards can affect the reading.
* Weigh yourself naked or remove shoes and heavy clothing.
* Stand weighing scales on a **solid floor**, not carpet.
* Weigh yourself on the same scales and the same floor surface at the same time of day.

Body mass index

Body mass index (BMI) is based upon height and weight so it doesn't take account of how much muscle you have. **Muscle is heavier than fat**; the more muscle you have, the heavier you are and the higher your BMI, yet you may not be **'overfat'**. Regular exercisers also have more muscle and weigh more.

To **calculate BMI**, divide weight (kg) by height (m^2) or input this information at http://www.eatwell.gov.uk/healthydiet/healthyweight/bmicalculator/ and it will calculate your BMI.

BMI of 18–24.9	Desirable
BMI of 25–30	Overweight
BMI of 30+	Obese
BMI of 40+	Morbidly obese

Tape measurements

Taking tape measurements is quick and easy, but can be inaccurate. Follow these guidelines for accurate measurements:

1 Take measurements on **bare skin** so clothes don't get in the way.
2 Measure at the **same place** – use 'body landmarks' such as the bellybutton for waist measurements and hip bones for hip measurements.
3 The **tape measure** should not be twisted, overtight or slack.
4 **Someone else taking the measurements** will give more accurate, less subjective measurements.
5 Note **dates and measurements** to track your monthly progress.

Although you can tighten muscle in specific areas, you **can't spot reduce body fat**, but you will lose different amounts from each area.

Waist–hip ratio

Measuring your **waist circumference** or **waist–hip ratio** will tell you if you are storing **fat around the middle** and provide an easy way to measure weight loss. **Fat around the middle** poses more of a **health risk** than fat around the thighs or bottom. It contributes to the development of **type 2 diabetes** and also increases production of low-density lipoprotein cholesterol ('bad' cholesterol) in the liver, which contributes to **coronary heart disease**. So, it is a good idea to keep your waist circumference within the guidelines given, and this provides an easy-to-measure goal for weight loss and improved health.

TOP TIP
View measurement-taking to calculate your **waist–hip ratio** at www.balancefood.ie/healthy-waist-and-hip-measurements/ or visit www.ashwell.uk.com/shapechart.pdf to **plot your waist measurement** on a chart.

Measuring your waist circumference:

* Locate the top of one hip bone and the bottom of the ribs on the same side.
* Halfway between is your waist – usually level with the navel/the narrowest part of your torso.

NHS waist circumference guidelines

Women	Men
Ideal: less than 80 cm (32 inches)	Ideal: less than 94 cm (37 inches)
High: 80–88 cm (32–35 inches)	High: 94–102 cm (37–40 inches)
Very high: more than 88 cm (35 inches)	Very high: more than 102 cm (40 inches)

The **waist–hip ratio** compares waist and hip circumference – the more **'apple' shaped** you are, the higher the level of associated health risks from **central obesity**.

Waist–hip ratio guidelines

Women	Men
Ideal: less than 0.8	Ideal: less than 0.9
Too high: 0.85 or more	Too high: 1 or more

To calculate your waist–hip ratio:

1 Measure your waist and hips in centimetres or inches.
2 Divide waist measurement by hip measurement as shown:
Waist: 80 cm; hips: 110 cm
Waist–hip ratio = 0.74.

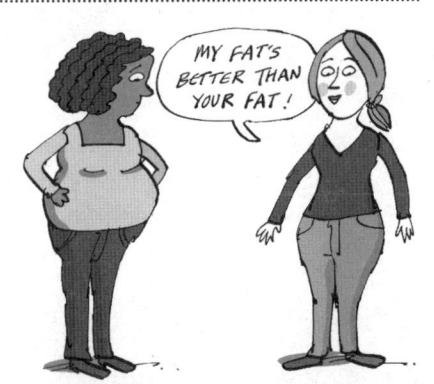

Body fat measurement

Body fat measurement devices send a light electrical current through the body, measuring the speed of the current through fat, muscle, bone and water. From this, estimates of water, muscle and fat proportions and weights are provided. **Hydration levels** (the amount of water in the body) affect the results, so you need to maintain adequate hydration for each measurement. Some weighing scales have **built-in impedance**, enabling you to measure total body weight and muscle and body fat levels.

Benefits

- ☑ Measuring body fat enables you to **check that the weight you are losing is mostly fat** and not lean tissue.
- ☑ If weight loss is slow, you can still see body fat levels reducing.

The type of body weight you want to lose is **fat**. Fad diets cause **water, glycogen or muscle loss,** which may look good on the scales, but **water and glycogen are regained** as soon as fluids and carbohydrates are consumed, and **muscle loss reduces metabolic rate.**

Measuring body fat helps you **lose the right type of weight**, though it may be slower than the drastic water, glycogen or muscle loss that some diets provide.

Whichever form of measurement you use, setting **realistic goals** will help you to achieve your goal and maintain it.

Reducing muscle tissue, glycogen or water weight for quick-fix weight loss are all counterproductive to long-term body fat reduction and weight loss

3 Setting a weight loss goal

A common mistake is failing to break up weight loss into **small steps**.

Benefits of mini weight loss goals:

1. Getting to your target weight is more **manageable**.
2. You can **celebrate success** along the way.
3. They help keep you **focused** and **on track**.

> **TOP TIP**
> A good **weight loss goal** is **5% of body weight**. Multiply weight in kilograms or pounds by 5, then divide by 100. For example: 148 lb × 5 = 740/100 = 7.4 lb

Your weight loss goal is not a limit – any extra weight lost over the goal set is a bonus!

Plan to lose this initial weight over **six weeks**. By dividing 5% of your body weight by six (weeks), you will have a **weekly weight loss goal**. For example, 7.4 lb divided by six weeks = 1.2 lb weight loss weekly.

Six weeks is a good time period for a **short-term goal** – not long enough to put off getting started, but long enough to achieve substantial weight loss. Remember, this is just your **first step** towards the total amount of weight you want to lose.

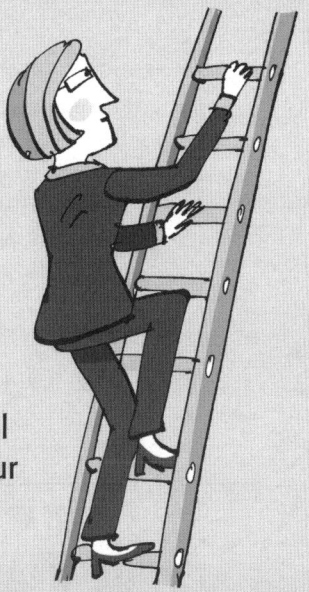

● Taking weight loss step by step is a successful strategy for long-term weight control

Weekly goals

If losing 5% of your current weight over six weeks means losing more than 2 lb weekly, you can either **limit your weekly weight loss goal to 2 lb** or **extend your deadline** to eight weeks. It's important to make weight loss goals **realistic** and **achievable** – many fad diets are based upon unachievable weight loss promises that end in failure and frustration, which often leads to overeating and regaining weight.

Common mistakes:

- ☒ trying to lose too much weight too quickly
- ☒ not breaking down the amount of weight you want to lose into smaller chunks.

It is better to take small steps in the right direction and get there eventually than to start off at a sprint but never arrive at the finish line

The **less you have to lose, the less fat you will lose** each week. If you have **a stone or less to lose**, aim to lose **0.5 lb** weekly – still a loss of almost half a stone over 12 weeks.

1–2 lb a week may not seem like a good weight loss, but with 3,500 calories in 1 lb of fat, you need to create a calorie deficit of approximately 7,000 calories a week – 1,000 calories a day – to lose just 2 lb a week!

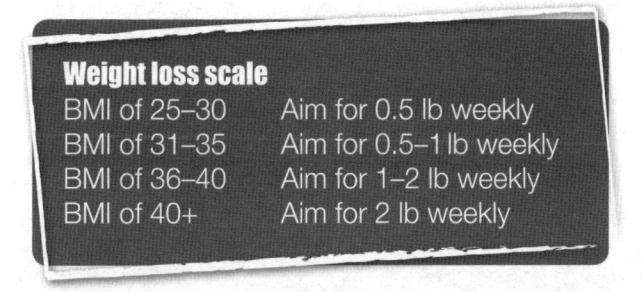

Weight loss scale

BMI of 25–30	Aim for 0.5 lb weekly
BMI of 31–35	Aim for 0.5–1 lb weekly
BMI of 36–40	Aim for 1–2 lb weekly
BMI of 40+	Aim for 2 lb weekly

SMART goals

Setting SMART goals for weight loss will increase your chance of success.

SMART stands for goals that are …

- **S**pecific
- **M**easurable
- **A**chievable
- **R**ealistic
- **T**ime bound.

SMART goals can significantly increase your chance of success

Setting your SMART weight loss goal

1. Choose a **specific** goal – weight loss, inch loss, reduced body fat percentage …
2. Your **measure** will be … weight on the scales, tape measurement, waist–hip ratio …
3. Your goal must be **achievable** and **realistic** – aiming to lose too much weight is likely to end in failure, which is demotivating and contributes to comfort eating and further weight gain.
4. Set a **date** to achieve it by. If you have an **event** that you would like to lose weight for, such as a wedding or holiday, you might want to use this date as your goal if it's within **four to eight weeks**.

Process vs outcome goals

Measuring weight loss by weighing yourself is an **outcome goal** – measuring the result rather than the **process** (what you do to achieve the goal). **Outcome-based goals are likely to be less successful than process-based goals** because …

* An outcome such as weight loss is not entirely in your **control**, it is **as a result of the process.**
* You have to wait to measure the outcome, so it lacks ongoing motivation.
* You have **control over process goals** – you can determine how many exercise minutes you complete, but you can't determine how much weight you lose.

Daily/weekly success of achieving a goal is likely to keep you motivated to stick with it as well as confirm that you are **on track for success.**

TOP TIP
Measure the journey, not the destination.

You can set yourself an **outcome goal** such as weight loss, plus a **process goal** to enable you to achieve the weight loss.

Examples of process goals:

* Complete 180 minutes of exercise each week.
* Limit alcohol consumption to 14 units per week.
* Reduce breakfast cereal portion size to 40 g, limit rice and pasta to 50 g.

You could set more than one process goal to help you achieve your weight loss, but limit yourself to a maximum of five to keep it simple and achievable.

If you have struggled to lose weight in the past, setting process goals and focusing on the journey rather than the destination could be the key to your success

Being realistic

Gauging whether your weight loss goal is **realistic** to achieve can be difficult at first. Take these things into consideration:

* How much do you weigh, and how much do you want to lose?
* Have you already lost weight?
* How much do you lose each week? Has it slowed down?
* How much exercise can you do?
* How much can you change your diet?

CASE STUDY

Cathie set a goal to lose one stone over six weeks and lost 8 lb. Failure to achieve the target led to comfort eating and weight gain. Then she planned to lose 6 lb over six weeks, lost 8 lb again, but overachieving her goal motivated her to continue. **The weight loss was the same, but the outcome completely different.**

It's important to **note your measurements** and **goal**, and the **date you will measure your success**. Write it in your diary, mark it on the calendar, maybe plan to treat yourself (not with chocolates!) when you reach your first goal weight.

Note down:

* your weight loss goal
* how you will achieve it (process goals like exercise minutes or dietary changes)
* the date you will achieve it by.

Telling others about your goal may also help, as you are more likely to set out to succeed and **meet other people's expectations** as well as your own. Now read on for tips on achieving that goal.

4 Fail to plan, plan to fail

Being organized and planning ahead will help you to succeed. Do you recognize these common dieting pitfalls?

* not having food in the house that is on the 'diet plan'
* having food in the house that is *not* on your 'diet plan'
* having to eat what is available
* letting yourself get **too hungry**
* not preparing **lunch** to take to work
* not planning time to **exercise**.

Sound familiar? If you've dieted before, you probably do recognise these hurdles that may have hindered your success.

Failing to plan is planning to fail

A good place to start is by completing a **food diary**. Simply write down everything that you eat and drink over a typical week, then look at it and decide what you will **change**. Following a strict diet usually ends in failure, but making small but effective changes to your current eating habits will result in success.

Identify things on your food diary that are contributing to weight gain, such as:

- biscuits, cakes, crisps, chocolate and sweets
- alcohol
- missing meals then snacking later
- big meals
- unnecessary bread with meals
- puddings
- high-calorie spreads, dips and sauces
- high-fat foods such as cheese.

Identify changes

Now that you've identified things that **contribute to weight gain**, decide what you will **change** – and **how** you will do it. Here are some suggestions:

- ☑ Reduce alcohol units from 14 to 7 per week.
- ☑ Replace cheese and biscuit snacks with fruit.
- ☑ Reduce 75 g of breakfast cereal to 40 g.
- ☑ Swap full-fat or semi-skimmed milk to skimmed milk.
- ☑ Drink water instead of fizzy drinks or juice.
- ☑ Stop eating bread with every meal.
- ☑ Replace high-calorie dips and sauces with low-calorie options.

You don't have to do all of these – just choose three or four things to work on. The next thing to do is **get organized**.

Plan ahead

Now that you've decided on the changes you will make, you need to ensure that you have the right foods in the house. Your next job is to **plan your meals** for the week ahead.

1. Make a food shopping list.
2. Buy the food you need – and don't buy foods that you are trying to avoid.
3. Prepare any meals in advance to make it easier to follow your plan and succeed.

> **TOP TIP**
> Don't go shopping when you are hungry – you are more likely to buy high-sugar, high-fat and higher calorie foods.

Shopping

A healthy eating week begins with **food shopping** – once you have biscuits or cakes at home, you will eat them.

Rule No. 1: Don't buy these foods!

Avoid confectionary and biscuit aisles in the supermarket – go shopping with a friend or partner who has your best interests at heart – he or she can step in when your **willpower** slips.

If temptation is too much, **shop online,** where you can't see the biscuits, smell the fresh bread or be drawn into buying two for one, or get someone else to shop for you.

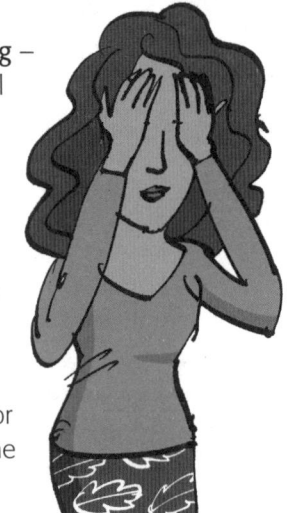

Out of sight, out of mind

If you buy crisps or cakes for others at home, put them in a cupboard you don't use often. Seeing them every time you open the usual cupboard is not helpful. You may go out and buy chocolate, but it's a hurdle that may be enough to deter you.

Other things that will help include:

* buying cakes, biscuits, chocolate or crisps that **you don't like**
* **freezing individual pieces** of cake, pies, or pudding to avoid having leftovers to hand
* freezing individual portions also means that they will require **defrosting** and should **limit you** to one serving
* **occupying your mind** at 'snacking' times by exercising, going out of the house or busying yourself with a hobby or work.

Treat yourself

Following a healthy diet to lose weight isn't all about what you can't eat – turn it on its head and **buy foods that you enjoy.**

- ☑ Buy exotic fruits for a tasty fruit salad.
- ☑ Buy prepared raw vegetables and low-fat dips for tasty snacks.
- ☑ Buy ready-made cartons of soup to make lunchtimes easy.
- ☑ Try new foods such as chickpeas, tofu, peppered mackerel or chillies.
- ☑ Try new recipes.

If you have fruit salad, soups or salads ready to eat, and dinner already planned, healthy eating is **easy**.

If you enjoy your new diet you are more likely to stick with it

Make it easy

To stick with your diet, it must be **easy to do**. Although this may mean more time planning and preparing meals, there are many ways of making it easier for yourself.

Rules for success

1. **One step at a time** – change just one or two things: when these are habitual, make more changes.
2. **Keep it simple** – have the same breakfast daily; buy soups for lunch; learn one new recipe a fortnight.
3. **Use leftovers** – make tomorrow's lunch with dinner.

Dinner	Lunch next day
Rice – cook an extra portion	Add salad for a cold rice salad
Baked potatoes – bake an extra one	Add salad for cold potato salad
Pasta – make an extra portion	Eat as it is or add salad for pasta salad

The plan

If you eat three meals daily, there are 21 meals that you can change to lose weight. Some of these will be easy to change, others more challenging.

You might want to start with the easiest for a quick win, or tackle the most problematic meals for greater weight loss.

Remember the bigger picture – total calorie intake versus total calorie expenditure – and balance higher calorie meals with lower calorie ones.

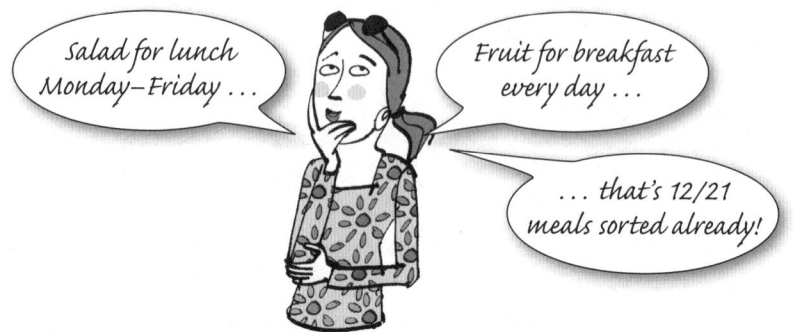

Salad for lunch Monday–Friday ...

Fruit for breakfast every day ...

... that's 12/21 meals sorted already!

Bullet Guide: Ten Rules for Guaranteed Weight Loss

Tools for success

Buying ready-made soups and salads **saves time**, but there are a number of other things that can help you to lose weight. If you have access to the **internet**, log on to any of these websites for tools such as:

* **food diaries** to print off or complete online
* **calorie or fat ready reckoners** to add up your daily intake
* BMI and waist circumference **calculators**
* **weight loss calculators** to help you plan and plot your weekly weight loss
* meal ideas and **recipes**
* ways of **measuring your success** – tot up exercise minutes or calorie intake.

www.weightlossresources.co.uk
www.tescodiets.com
www.weightconcern.org.uk
www.bdaweightwise.com

5 Reducing calorie intake

Most people cut out **calories** to lose weight, but most diets only last as long as their **willpower** – experts reckon between three days and three weeks! When people diet, they exclude all high-calorie/high-fat/sweet foods, which is initially effective, but difficult to stick to and short lived.

The good news is that you can **choose** what to cut out, and which foods to limit or swap for lower calorie alternatives.

You don't have to cut out everything ... just make enough changes to create a calorie deficit

However, knowing what to cut out and actually doing it are two different things! A good way to start is to write down everything you eat and drink, then highlight things to change. There is no food that you have to cut out completely, or for ever – successful **weight control** is about making choices:

* Which foods will you avoid?
* Which foods will you limit?
* Which foods can you change to a lower calorie option?

The more changes you make, the bigger the calorie deficit and the greater the weight loss.

Identify targets

High-calorie foods

First you need to identify high-calorie foods that you eat regularly:

* cakes
* biscuits
* chocolate
* sweets
* ice cream
* puddings and desserts
* full-fat dairy products
* spreads, dips and oils
* fatty meats
* nuts
* alcohol.

You can check the calorie content of foods at www.weightlossresources.co.uk.

If you consume more calories than you use up, you will gain weight – it's as simple as that!

Reducing quantities

You might cut out some foods, but just limit others. Although this may not reduce your calorie intake as much, you'll **stick with it for longer**, losing more weight in the long run. Look at your **food diary** and decide what to tackle first – things such as:

1 limiting the units of alcohol you drink in a week
2 sharing a pudding if you eat out
3 having **one biscuit** with your cup of tea, **not two**
4 buying **lower calorie** dips and spreads
5 eating **smaller** chocolate bars.

> **TOP TIP**
> Make a few changes that you can stick with, then, once these are habitual, revisit your list and make more changes.

Lower calorie foods

You can also choose to eat **lower calorie versions** of foods that you commonly eat, such as:

* changing full-fat or semi-skimmed milk to skimmed milk
* choosing low-fat yoghurts
* using low-fat spreads, sauces and dips
* eating lower calorie foods or meals.

● Reduced calorie foods can leave you feeling less satisfied than the higher calorie versions, causing you to eat more of them and ending up with the same calorie intake! Don't slip up by thinking that diet foods can be eaten freely – we often need to change our eating **habits** rather than our **food choices**

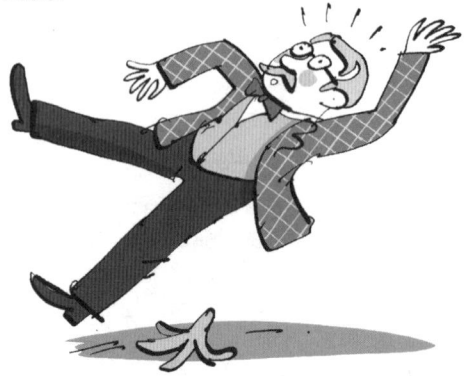

Bullet Guide: Ten Rules for Guaranteed Weight Loss

Change your thinking

Change thought processes from 'Just a mouthful won't make a difference' into '**Every mouthful makes a difference**'. Once you are looking for ways to **reduce calorie intake**, you will begin to **stop yourself** pinching a crisp, finishing the children's leftover chips, having a biscuit, saying 'yes' to another bread roll … because **it does all add up**.

Remember, just to lose 1 lb a week requires a **deficit of approximately 500 calories** each day. Get into the habit of jotting down all the ways you have reduced your calorie intake daily – you'll then be more likely to say 'no' to a biscuit because you can add it to your list!

CASE STUDY

Amanda made one change to her diet every few weeks. Weight loss was steady rather than dramatic, but she didn't feel like she was dieting, and could stick with her new eating plan, ultimately achieving her target weight.

Change your behaviour

Eating behaviours are to blame for many an expanding waistline. Do you recognize any of these habits?

- eating out of **habit** at certain times of the day when you're not even hungry
- eating out of **boredom**
- **comfort eating** to make yourself feel better
- eating something simply because it **goes with something else**, such as always having a biscuit with a cup of tea
- eating just because someone else is, e.g. dessert.

If so, you will benefit from changing your **eating behaviour**. If you can **identify why** you eat certain foods and **change the circumstance**, you won't have to rely on your willpower.

Change how you eat, not what you eat

Bullet Guide: Ten Rules for Guaranteed Weight Loss

- Although eating late is not generally recommended, if you eat dinner early and then snack later on, eating dinner later on may **stop you snacking** and reduce your evening calorie intake.
- We often consume certain things together (**food association**). If you can't have a cup of tea or coffee without biscuits, change your drinking habits instead of trying not to have biscuits. Herbal teas or cold drinks don't need biscuits on the side.
- **Don't get hungry**. When blood sugar levels drop you crave foods high in sugar or calories. If you eat regularly throughout the day, you can **remove physiological cravings** for sugary foods.
- Drink plenty of water throughout the day so that you **don't mistake thirst for hunger**.

Avoid triggers

There are times when we are **more likely to overeat**, so avoiding these circumstances will help you to limit your calorie intake:

1 buffets
2 eating off larger plates
3 eating while doing something else, such as watching television.

Satiety – the feeling of fullness – is specific to the food we are 'full' of, leaving us able to 'find space' for desserts after a large meal, or graze all night at a buffet. Eat before you go out and avoid the buffet table!

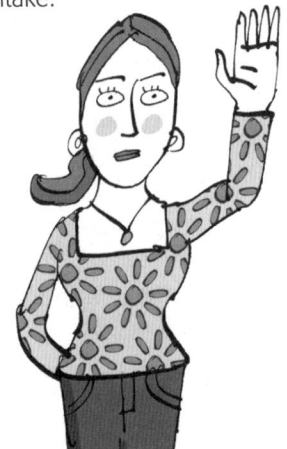

● Stop and think before you approach the buffet table!

Bullet Guide: Ten Rules for Guaranteed Weight Loss

Top tips for reducing calorie consumption

1. Swap to skimmed milk or black tea/coffee.
2. Drink less alcohol.
3. Say 'no' to the bread basket.
4. Pack out meals with lower calorie fruit and vegetables.
5. Swap fizzy drinks and juices for no-calorie water.

These are just options … make a list of everything you could change and choose one or two things at a time rather than trying to do it all at once. Jumping from where you are to 'optimum nutrition' in one go will result in failure – better to **take one step at a time**, reach your destination and stay there, rather than diet again and again.

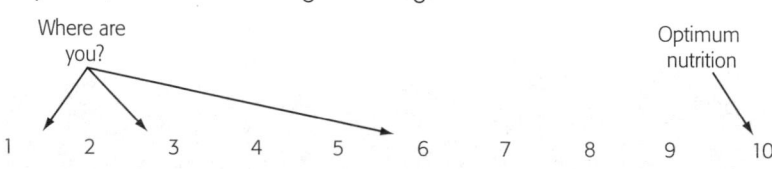

Where are you? → 2, 3, 6

Optimum nutrition → 10

1 2 3 4 5 6 7 8 9 10

6 Portion control

If you have already reduced **high-calorie foods** in your diet, but are still not losing weight, you may be **eating too much**. But how much is too much?

A portion is the size of the palm of your hand. A healthy meal includes the following portions:

* one of protein (fish, eggs, meat, dairy or pulses)
* one of starchy carbohydrates (rice, pasta, etc.)
* one or two of non-starch polysaccharide (fruit or vegetables).

Regardless of the type of foods you eat, if you eat too much in one go, you will convert excess calories into body fat

Although **portion control** is important for all foods, we are most likely to **overeat carbohydrate-rich foods** such as bread, pasta or cereals. It's time consuming to weigh everything you eat, but **controlling the amount of starchy carbohydrates** in your diet could be a breakthrough in your efforts to lose weight.

Recommended carbohydrate portion sizes:

Cereals	30–40 g
Rice	50–75 g
Pasta	50–75 g
Bread	One or two slices
Potatoes	One medium-sized potato

Why do we overeat?

Just as 'if you buy it, you eat it', where portion size is concerned **'if you serve it, you eat it'**. There are many **reasons why we overeat**:

1. We like the taste of the food so **continue to eat past satiety**.
2. We don't want to **waste food**.
3. We habitually **ignore body signals to stop eating**.
4. We tend to overeat when we have **missed meals** or **reduced calorie intake too much**, so graze through the day to avoid getting too hungry.

> **TOP TIP**
> Weigh the amount of rice or cereal you usually have. Make no change if it is less than the suggested amounts – otherwise, reduce it. Reducing 80 g of starchy carbohydrates to 40 g could save you about 150 calories each meal.

Change your behaviour

Food preparation

Food preparation can be easier to change than eating behaviour – if you don't prepare too much food in the first place, you are less likely to overeat, so changes in eating behaviour begins with food preparation:

1 Weigh out food so you don't cook more than you need.
2 Remember that the more different foods there are in a meal, the less of each you need.

To help you get used to eating smaller portions ...

- ☑ **Eat slowly** – this makes the meal last longer and gives your body time to create the feeling of satiety.
- ☑ **Don't do other things while you eat** or you are more likely to eat quickly.
- ☑ **Take a sip of water** or **put down your knife and fork** between mouthfuls.
- ☑ **Chew** each mouthful thoroughly.

Use smaller plates

If a meal looks small you are likely to want to eat more afterwards, so **using smaller plates and dishes** helps a smaller portion to look like a plateful.

Reduce calories, not meal size

A **full plate** is less likely to leave you feeling hungry, even if the calorie content is lower, so replace calorie-dense foods such as pasta or cereal with **lower calorie vegetables or fruit.**

Having a **full plate of food** makes you feel as if you are not 'on a diet'. Fruits and vegetables contain lots of fibre and water – there are no calories in water and very few available to us in fibre. These make your meal look larger and also make you feel full.

What to reduce	What to add in
Cereal	Fruit – berries, citrus fruits, apple, pear, melon, apricot, mango
Pasta	Water-rich aubergines, courgettes, red onions, garlic, tomatoes …
Potatoes	Any other vegetables – pumpkin, carrot, beetroot, broccoli …
Rice	Make risotto with onions, garlic, frozen peas, peppers and sweetcorn or add extra vegetables to chilli, curry or stroganoff
Proteins/fats	Use fewer eggs in omelettes but add tomatoes, peppers, onion, rocket … Have a smaller meat or fish portion and fill up on lower calorie vegetables Serve wafer-thin cheese but lots of salad vegetables

Remember, you are **replacing** one food with another, not just adding fruit or vegetables! To control calorie intake, if you increase the amount of one food on your plate (e.g. fruit), you have to reduce another (e.g. cereal).

'Eat until you are 80% full.'

Learn when to stop

Even with all these tips, if you have a healthy appetite, you need to change your **eating behaviour** if you want to lose weight and keep it off. You must learn how to:

* **stop eating** when you begin to feel full
* **leave food** on your plate
* **refrigerate or freeze** leftover food rather than have another serving
* **throw leftovers away** so that you don't starting eating again later.

TOP TIP
See how much food is left on your plate when you begin to feel full – this is the amount you have overprepared. Next time you prepare this meal, reduce your portion size by the amount of food left over rather than rely on willpower to stop eating.

Limit the foods in a meal

Eating too many different foods in one meal is likely to result in **overeating** as we are less likely to become bored with one food and continue to eat.

The feeling of satiety is specific: we decide we have eaten enough of one food but will continue to consume other foods. This is experienced when eating out – we may feel 'full' and wouldn't eat another plate of lasagne, for example, but will gladly order dessert.

We are also likely to overeat when there are a lot of different foods on our plate, so keep meals simple with fewer ingredients and this may help you to reduce calorie intake.

To ensure you do **reduce overall calorie count** when replacing calorie-rich foods with other foods:

1 **Don't add too many foods to a meal** – replace starchy carbohydrates with equivalent portion sizes of fruit or vegetables.
2 To ensure you get it right, **weigh foods**.

If you are reducing a cereal portion by 25 g, just add 25 g of fruit.

If you are reducing your rice portion by 50 g, add 50 g of vegetables.

As fruit and vegetables (non-starch polysaccharides) contain less starch but more water than starchy carbohydrates, although the food weight remains the same, non-starch polysaccharides contain fewer calories. For example, 89% of carrots is water (no calories), whereas only 11.4% of white rice is water.

A plan for life

For a weight loss plan that works for life, keep an eye on your **portion sizes**. Remember …

* **Prepare less food** – you can always snack later if you haven't had enough to eat, but, if you prepare too much, you will eat it whether you need it or not.
* **Fill your plate with lower calorie foods** such as fruit or vegetables – a plateful of food will make you feel fuller.
* **Eat slowly** – and **stop eating** once you feel full.
* Remember, **satiety is specific** – a smorgasbord of food leads to higher calorie intake, so keep meals simple.

And the golden rule … limit the overall size of each meal.

It's not what you eat, it's how much you eat that matters!

7 Increasing calorie expenditure

Healthy eating plus regular exercise = successful weight loss. In addition to expending calories while exercising, your **metabolism** stays elevated afterwards, and, if you build **muscle**, you will boost metabolism and use more calories whether you are exercising, working or sleeping.

Remember the energy balance equation …

> … if calories in are less than calories out, you lose weight.

So increasing calorie expenditure is just as effective as reducing calorie intake – if you do both, you'll lose weight twice as fast.

The more active you are, the more you can get away with eating!

Regular exercise is the most effective way to **use calories**, but just being more **active** will help create a **calorie deficit**. Try these:

- Use the stairs, not the lift.
- Try to walk around every half hour – go and speak to colleagues instead of sending emails!
- Leave the car at home and walk to the shops or school.
- Get off the bus, tube or train a stop early.
- Start an active hobby such as dancing or gardening.
- Take the dog (or someone else's dog) for a walk.
- Do the housework – it contributes to calorie expenditure!

What type of exercise?

Cardiovascular exercise uses more calories – the most effective 'calorie-burning exercises' are **higher intensity** and **weight-bearing** exercises such as running, hillwalking or fitness classes. Weight-bearing exercise is when you support your body weight.

Compare weight-bearing (shaded) and non-weight-bearing exercises …

Activity	Approximate calories/hour
Running (7.5 miles/hour)	697
High-impact aerobics	414
Rowing at moderate intensity	365
Cycling (10 miles/hour)	305
Swimming (recreational)	250

Compiled from information available at www.weightlossresources.co.uk

Cycling, rowing or swimming are **non-weight-bearing exercises** because your body weight is supported: although still beneficial, you have to work harder to use the same number of calories as in a weight-bearing exercise.

Weight training is a weight-bearing exercise because of the resistance applied against the muscles. Although weight training may increase the amount of muscle you have, and may therefore increase your overall body weight by a little, the overall effect will reduce **body fat** levels, as the more muscle you have, the higher your **metabolic rate** is. This means that you will use up more calories, whatever you are doing, over a 24 hour period. Gaining lean tissue helps to turn your body into a **fat-burning machine!**

For every extra pound of muscle you put on, your body uses around 50 extra calories a day.

Juliette Kellow, Weight Loss Resources

How much exercise?

How much exercise you need to do depends on how much weight you want to lose. To lose 1 lb a week, you need a **calorie deficit** of 500 calories a day.

The harder the exercise, the less time you need to spend doing it – you would need to walk quickly for almost 2 hours to use up approximately 500 calories, but you could expend the same energy in a 45 minute run, although **calorie usage** depends upon weight, body composition and fitness level.

Workouts that would use up approximately 500 calories:

* one hour high-intensity dance or aerobics class
* 45 minutes on a step machine in the gym
* one hour playing a reasonably hard game of tennis
* one hour of cycling.

The more **effort** you put in, the greater the rewards. However, most people exercise at a level that feels comfortable, without getting out of breath or sweating too much.

> **TOP TIP**
> To know if you are working hard enough to make a difference, you should exercise at a **perceived exertion rate** of 7–8 on a scale of 1–10.

As your body becomes accustomed to the exercise, you will use fewer calories, so, to continue losing weight, continue to increase the **intensity** so it never becomes too easy.

As you lose weight you use fewer calories doing the same exercise, which can stall your **weight loss**. Exercising harder or longer, or changing the exercise session, will maximize exercise calorie utilization.

How long?

Having no time is a **common excuse** for not exercising, but even 20 minutes' exercise will expend calories, increase **metabolic rate** and help create an **exercise habit**. The longer you exercise, and/or the harder you work, the more calories you use.

When we start to exercise we use more **carbohydrate energy**. As time progresses, we use more **fat** in our **'fuel mix'**. Longer duration activities are therefore referred to as **'fat burning'**. However, they are also usually lower intensity so calorie expenditure is not automatically higher.

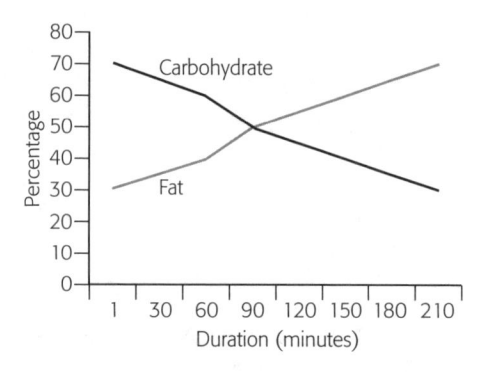

● Percentage carbohydrate and fat used during exercise

Bullet Guide: Ten Rules for Guaranteed Weight Loss

How hard?

Interval training, whereby higher intensity exercise is alternated with easier phases, aids weight loss. During the **higher intensity phases** you utilize more calories than usual, and the easier phases allow you to **recover**. You wouldn't do an entire workout at the higher intensity, but working harder in **spurts** will burn more calories yet enable you to do a longer workout.

Creating an interval training session	As you get fitter …
Jog 1 minute, walk 1 minute	Increase time jogging, decrease time walking
Cycle faster 2 minutes, cycle slowly 1 minute	Increase faster cycling or cycle uphill
Swim one length quickly, swim back slowly	Do more faster lengths

The most important thing about exercise is to make it a **regular** occurrence!

Get the habit

To lose weight and keep it off you need to create an **exercise habit**. **Exercise dissociation** such as **exercising with others** or **listening to music** takes your mind off the exercise you are doing and relieves boredom and exercise discomfort …

It also makes exercise more **enjoyable** and **sociable**, and reduces the likelihood of missing an exercise session if you are letting someone else down. It is essential that you find something that you enjoy doing – if you don't **enjoy** it, you won't keep it up.

You are more likely to continue exercising if you exercise with others

Bullet Guide: Ten Rules for Guaranteed Weight Loss

Motivate yourself

Set yourself an **exercise goal**. This is known as a **process goal**, as you are measuring the process rather than relying on an **outcome goal** such as weight loss. For example …

'I will do two exercise sessions each week' or 'I will do 600 exercise minutes each month'.

For a successful exercise plan:

1. Choose exercise you enjoy.
2. Unless self-motivated, **exercise with others.**
3. Choose weight-bearing, higher intensity activities to expend more calories.
4. Use **interval training** and keep your overall perceived exertion rate over 6.
5. Set exercise goals.

… and if all else fails, and you simply can't motivate yourself to exercise regularly, get a personal trainer!

8 Manipulating protein and carbohydrate intake

Carbohydrate foods affect our **blood sugar** the most as they contain starches and sugars that may be absorbed into the bloodstream quickly. Foods with a **high glycaemic index (GI)** contain more glucose (a simple sugar); foods with a **low GI** contain less readily available glucose and provide a more sustained energy release rather than a quick 'high'.

Carbohydrate-rich foods
- Potatoes
- Rice
- Beans and pulses
- Breakfast cereals
- Bread
- Pasta

Low-carbohydrate diets are a popular way of losing weight, but there are pros and cons. Carbohydrates are essential for health, providing energy, fibre and essential nutrients, so carbohydrate intake should not be less than **50–60% of total calorie intake**.

Weight loss on low-carbohydrate diets is often due to **reduced glycogen (stored glucose) and water**, which return as soon as carbohydrates are eaten. A low-carbohydrate diet will also leave you **lacking energy** and unlikely to exercise.

However, there are ways you can **adjust your carbohydrate intake to boost weight loss** and achieve long-term weight maintenance.

Use the GI scale to choose slow-release carbohydrates over 'quick fix' sugars

Controlling blood sugar

Low-fat diets are common, as fat contains the most calories per gram. However, low-fat 'diet' foods often contain lots of **sugar,** which affects successful weight control. Although carbohydrates contain fewer calories than fats, they can be detrimental to our eating habits:

* When blood sugar is low we crave sugary, fatty and higher calorie foods.
* Carbohydrate-rich foods are often **'trigger' foods** that we overeat, such as bread, chocolate, pasta or biscuits.
* Too much sugar in the bloodstream makes us produce a hormone called **insulin**, which can be detrimental to long-term weight control.

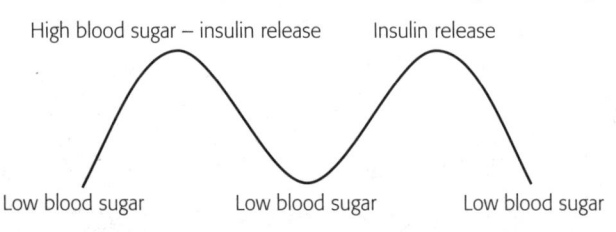

High blood sugar – insulin release   Insulin release

Low blood sugar   Low blood sugar   Low blood sugar

Glycaemic index

The **glycaemic index (GI)** is a scale of 1–100, indicating how quickly and how much glucose in foods is absorbed into the bloodstream.

* Low GI: food has low glucose content or contains mostly starches.
* High GI: food contains more glucose for a quick energy surge.

High GI Food	GI	Lower GI Alternative	GI
Parsnips	97	Cauliflower	0
White baguette	95	Rye bread	51
Easy-cook white rice	87	Brown rice	55
Rice pudding	81	Fruit yoghurt	33
Watermelon	72	Grapefruit	25
Puffed wheat	80	Porridge	49
White bread	70	Oat cakes	54
Chocolate ice cream	68	Strawberry mousse	32
Fizzy orange drink	68	Apple juice	40

High GI (70 and above – black shading); medium GI (55–70 – grey shading); low GI (below 55 – no shading).

Although the **GI** indicates whether a food contains a high proportion of glucose in relation to other sugars, not all high GI foods contain large amounts of glucose. For example, watermelon has a high GI, but a typical portion contains only 14 g of carbohydrate (compare this with 40 g in a 250 ml bottle of Lucozade) – it's mostly water.

The **glycaemic load (GL)** of a food gives values according to the **blood glucose effect** of a **normal portion** of the food or drink.

GL = (GI × weight (g) of carbohydrate to be eaten)/100

The higher the carbohydrate grams per portion in a food, the higher the GL, and, if the carbohydrate is mostly glucose, it will be absorbed quickly and elevate blood sugar.

Riper fruits and vegetables will have a higher GI – a ripe banana contains more sugars than a starchy green banana

If we eat **quick-release (high GI) carbohydrates** that elevate blood sugar (blood glucose), **insulin** reduces the glucose in our bloodstream:

1. It increases cellular glucose absorption.
2. It increases the glucose stored as glycogen.
3. It **reduces fat breakdown** for energy so that we can use excess glucose.
4. It stimulates **conversion of excess glucose into fat**.

High-carbohydrate intake prompts increased insulin release, and the more insulin we release, the lower the resulting blood sugar level is, making us crave more sugar or quick-release carbohydrates.

> *High insulin levels contribute to obesity, so although sugary/high GI foods may not be high in calories, these foods are not good for the waistline.*

The **GI** of foods can help you to lose weight because:

1. It helps you to identify foods rich in sugars or starch.
2. It helps you to balance your blood sugar level and reduce insulin release.
3. This enables you to limit conversion of sugars into fat.

Dieting is often counter-productive to weight loss as the calorie reduction leaves you hungry, so you end up eating just as much or more than usual in an attempt to elevate blood sugar. Using the GI will enable you to **avoid low blood sugar levels** so that you don't have to rely on your willpower to stop you eating sugary/fatty foods.

Every dieter knows that the diet goes out the window when hunger sets in!

High-fibre foods

Eating **high-fibre** carbohydrates slows down the release of glucose into the bloodstream, aiding **blood glucose control**. Swap high GI foods for higher fibre, lower GI options:

- ☑ Swap white bread for wholemeal or GI bread.
- ☑ Swap white rice for brown rice.
- ☑ Swap white pasta for wholewheat pasta.
- ☑ Replace potatoes with broccoli, cabbage or salad.

Weighing the portion size of cereal, rice or pasta will also help you to reduce your carbohydrate intake and insulin production.

Cereal portion	30–40 g
Uncooked rice or pasta portion	50–75 g

High-protein foods

You can also **reduce the GI of a meal by including protein foods at each mealtime**, which helps to slow down carbohydrate digestion and glucose absorption. Another benefit of eating protein foods is that they make us **feel full**, reducing the likelihood of eating sugary snacks between meals.

Combining protein foods with low GI carbohydrates:

- ☑ porridge oats with yoghurt
- ☑ peppered mackerel with chickpea and mixed bean salad
- ☑ brown rice with chicken, turkey, fish or tofu.

To use the best elements of popular 'high-protein, low-carbohydrate' diets:

* Reduce your intake of high GI, refined carbohydrates.
* Eat low GI, high-fibre whole foods.
* Eat protein with each meal.

Manipulating the GI of your meals

- ☑ Avoid or limit **refined carbohydrates** with a high GI.
- ☑ Eat **smaller portions** of high GI foods.
- ☑ **Combine** high GI foods with low GI foods.
- ☑ Eat **high-fibre** carbohydrates to limit GI.
- ☑ **Eat protein** with each meal to slow down glucose absorption and avoid blood sugar highs and lows.
- ☑ Eat **al dente vegetables**, which take longer to digest.

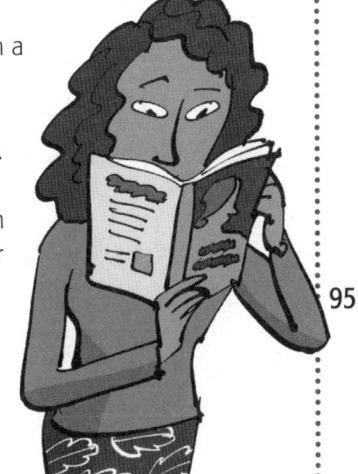

● Use a GI counter book to create a low GI diet

9 Jumping over hurdles for long-term success

If your social life is affecting your weight loss, it's time to take control. You can still enjoy yourself, but employing **'damage limitation'** and not going 'all out' on every social occasion will deliver the results you are after.

If you find it difficult to …

… **limit** calorie intake

… **employ moderation** when eating out

… **maintain** your weight over Christmas or while on holiday …

then you need a damage limitation plan!

The things you want to eat will still be there tomorrow… there's no need to eat them all in one go!

Bullet Guide: Ten Rules for Guaranteed Weight Loss

Ideally, you should be able to relax and enjoy a meal out, choosing to eat whatever you want, but if you **overindulge** too often, you won't achieve your weight loss goals.

Trying to opt for **lower calorie options** or eat healthily when eating out can be very difficult:

1 A dish might appear to be low calorie but when it arrives it may be covered in a **high-fat/high-calorie sauce or dressing**.
2 Most restaurant meals use more **butter, oil, cheese and other fats** in their dishes than you would at home, enhancing flavour but also calorie count.

Eating out

The more often you eat out, the more you need to use these tips to limit calorie intake:

* Drink **still or sparking water** instead of juice or alcohol.
* Order salads but **hold the dressing** or put it **on the side.**
* **Avoid snacking** on bar and table appetizers such as salted nuts and breadsticks.
* Ignore the bread basket!
* Choose broth or vegetable-based, rather than cream-based, **soups**.
* Choose low-fat vegetarian, fish or lean meat options.
* Ask about dishes and **see if the chef can modify your meal** by serving sauces and dressings on the side, or leaving cheese out of a dish or cream off dessert.

Tips to limit calorie intake

* **Don't starve yourself all day** if you're going out for dinner – you are likely to choose options higher in fat, sugar and calories and eat more if you are **overhungry**.
* **Order a starter** as a main meal, or a second starter in place of a main meal.
* **Order a children's meal** – the portion size is likely to be smaller.
* **Share a pudding** – you'll be doing your pudding partner a favour too as you halve the portion and halve the calories.
* Order a coffee instead of dessert.

● Check menus carefully for the lowest calorie option

Alcohol

Alcohol can be the ruin of many a good diet! Pure alcohol provides **seven calories per gram** – just a little less than fats, and as its liquid it's easy to consume a large amount without feeling full. A couple of glasses of wine in the evenings are counter-productive to weight loss.

> An *alcohol unit* depends upon the *alcohol volume*, but is generally *half a pint* of standard-strength beer, lager or cider, or a *measure of spirits*, and a *glass of wine is usually two units*. It is recommended that women don't exceed *14 units* a week and men stay within *21 units* a week for good health.

As with any aspect of your diet, you don't need to cut out alcohol completely unless you want to.

Bullet Guide: Ten Rules for Guaranteed Weight Loss

Tips to reduce alcohol intake

- Limit weekly alcohol units.
- Have alcohol-free days.
- Drink spritzers, which last longer than wine.
- Alternate alcoholic drinks with mineral water.
- Swap wine for alcohol-free wine, or dilute red or white grape juice with water.
- Arrive late and miss the first round, or, if drinking at home, start later! If you have drunk a large part of a bottle of wine by the time you eat dinner, you'll end up opening a second bottle.
- Don't go out thirsty – the first couple of drinks won't touch the sides!
- Drive, don't drink!

Limiting your alcohol intake could be the only thing you need to do to tip the scales in your favour

Holidays

Many people gain weight on holiday, but you can still employ 'damage limitation' while away, and the break from routine might even help you to follow different eating and exercise habits.

Follow these tips to come back lighter:

* **Don't overindulge in everything all at once** – no need to have ice-cream *and* pudding *and* cocktails every day!
* Don't book **all-inclusive holidays** – they are a temptation to overeat.
* **Drink water through the day** rather than alcohol, juices, fizzy drinks and cocktails.
* Eat lots of healthy fish and salad.
* Keep up the good habits you follow at home.
* Don't add unnecessary bread to your meals.

How to survive the buffet meal or all-inclusive resort ...

- ☑ Use smaller plates.
- ☑ Don't add sauces and dips.
- ☑ **Eat slowly** and savour your meal.
- ☑ Fill your plate with fruit or salad vegetables.
- ☑ If you want to taste a few different things, **take smaller amounts**.
- ☑ **Choose either** a starter and main meal OR a main meal and dessert.
- ☑ Many dishes at all-inclusive buffets are repeated – **you don't have to have everything** every day.
- ☑ **Don't eat for the sake of it** – if dessert doesn't look appetizing, don't have it.

Christmas

Most people **gain weight over Christmas** – but to avoid spending half the year losing the weight you've gained:

* **Keep exercising** – even though you have Christmas shopping, present wrapping and writing cards to do, make sure you find time to offset those additional Christmas calories!
* Employ **damage limitation** at Christmas parties and buffets.
* Have a couple of **mini-detox days** before and after Christmas to offset the higher calorie intake – you'll feel much better for eating nothing but fruit, vegetables and water for a day.

Detox plan

Breakfast	Hot water with lime/lemon; fruit salad and freshly squeezed fruit juice
Lunch	Vegetable soup or salad
Dinner	Vegetable stir fry

Plenty of water throughout the day

Yuletide tips to avoid feeling stuffed

- Eat a little of everything for Christmas dinner, but **keep overall meal size small.**
- Limit starchy carbohydrates – have one type of potato.
- Eat slowly and stop when you feel full.
- Alternate **alcoholic drinks** with sparkling water, or only drink with dinner.
- Don't put chocolates or nuts out to nibble at all day.
- Have **Christmas pudding later** to reduce lunchtime calories.
- Have Greek yoghurt or crème fraiche **instead of cream** with Christmas pudding.

… and hopefully you'll see the year out weighing less than you weighed in January, not needing a 'new year, new you' diet!

10 A diet for life

How many times have you lost weight but failed to keep it off? **Slimming clubs** are full of people **'yo-yo-ing'** between fat and thin wardrobes. If this sounds familiar, and you want to **stop dieting**, you need a long-term approach enabling you to **stay within 7 lb of your target weight**, so you never have to 'diet' again …

1. It has to be **enjoyable** otherwise you won't stick to it.
2. Calories in must equal calorie expenditure for **weight maintenance**.
3. It has to be sustainable for **health**.

For long-term success, you need a 'diet for life'

As well as **balancing calories** so calories in equal calories out, a long-term, sustainable healthy diet needs all the nutrients essential for good health – it needs to tick all these boxes:

- ☑ At least **five portions of fruit and vegetables** daily.
- ☑ **Two to three portions of protein** (fish, meat, dairy products, eggs or soya products) daily.
- ☑ **Starchy carbohydrates** in two to three meals daily.
- ☑ Eight glasses of **water** daily.
- ☑ **Limit** saturated fats, salt, sugar and processed foods.

Diets excluding entire food groups are not long-term healthy eating plans – and if you can't follow a diet for life, what happens when you come 'off' it?

Balancing calories

Balancing calories for life doesn't have to mean weighing foods, counting calories or points – you just need to keep an eye on overall calorie intake and expenditure – the **big picture** rather than individual meals.

Tips for success

- ☑ Eat high-calorie foods occasionally not daily.
- ☑ **Weigh** rice, pasta and cereals and limit bread.
- ☑ **Offset** big meals and blowout weekends with leaner meals or detox weekends.
- ☑ **Do more exercise** to counteract times when you have eaten more.

Events such as holidays, Christmas and job changes will test you throughout life, and you must be able to survive these challenges by **adjusting your calorie intake and expenditure** accordingly.

Keeping track

Extra pounds don't appear overnight – you put them there by consuming too many calories or not being active enough. By keeping an eye on your weight, you can **take action** and avoid going back to square one with an **early intervention plan**!

1. Set a weight or measurement range to stay within.
2. Check measurements monthly.
3. If you notice your waistband expanding or clothes feeling tight, **act immediately**.

> Remember, there are 3,500 calories in 1 lb of fat, so a loss of 4 lb requires a calorie deficit of 14,000 calories! It already sounds monumental – no wonder it can take years to reduce body weight by a couple of stones.

Getting back on track

- **Limit high-calorie foods and drinks** such as alcohol, biscuits, cakes, chocolate, ice cream, sauces, fatty meats, sausages and burgers.
- **Weigh** out cereals, rice and pasta.
- **Limit** bread and potatoes.
- **Reduce portion sizes** – it may not be what you're eating but how much.
- **Snack on raw vegetables or fruit** instead of biscuits, cakes or crisps.
- Do more **exercise** – or work harder at it.
- **Repeat the things you did** to reduce your body weight initially!

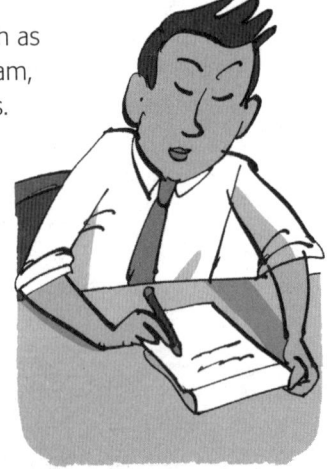

● If you begin to gain weight, get back on track with an early intervention plan

Keeping active

If you are consuming the right amount of calories but are **still gaining weight**, or still need to lose weight, try concentrating on **using up more energy** through increased activity levels and exercise rather than reducing your calorie intake any further.

Remember, if you reduce your calorie intake below that needed to sustain your basal metabolic rate, you run the risk of reducing your **metabolism**. This will lead to gains in body fat and make it difficult for you to lose weight. Exercising, however, will help you to increase your **metabolic rate**.

'Regular exercise is an essential part of any successful long-term weight loss strategy.'

Increasing exercise intensity

- ☑ Exercise for longer and more frequently.
- ☑ **Work harder** – run faster, swim faster, cycle harder.
- ☑ **Change** your gym programme.
- ☑ Try a **new or harder** exercise class.
- ☑ Graduate from walking to **hillwalking.**
- ☑ **Carry a rucksack** with water bottles or other weights in it.
- ☑ **Reduce rest time** when you exercise.

TOP TIP

As you lose weight, try to counteract the reduced calorie expenditure by carrying the equivalent body weight lost in a weighted vest or rucksack – this will enable you to burn more calories per exercise session, but is most useful for activities such as walking.

Bullet Guide: Ten Rules for Guaranteed Weight Loss

Making lifestyle changes

Increasing **activity levels** throughout the day can **tip the scales** in your favour, and you are likely to stick with **lifestyle changes** once they are habitual. You are unlikely to exercise for even one hour every day, but can maximize calorie expenditure in the remaining 23 hours with a few simple changes:

- ☑ Take the **stairs** not the lift.
- ☑ **Walk** to work, school, college, the shops …
- ☑ Take the dog for a **walk.**
- ☑ **Walk** on your lunch break.
- ☑ **Busy yourself** around the house and garden.
- ☑ **Get a pedometer** and set daily step goals.

Setting goals

It may help you to succeed if you **set goals** or plan **rewards** through the year …

Date	Goal	Plan	Reward
14 February	Lose 6 lb	180 exercise minutes weekly No alcohol	Valentine's weekend away
1 April	Lose 4 lb	Three classes weekly Stick to eating plan	Birthday meal out
14 May	Lose 2 lb	Three classes weekly Reduce portion sizes	Go clothes shopping
1 July	Lose 2 lb – reach target weight	Alcohol units to three per week Salads for lunch	Go on holiday
14 August	Lose 2 lb gained on holiday	220 exercise minutes weekly	New dress for barbeque
1 October	Maintain goal weight	Swap swim for gym Yoga twice weekly to tone up	Spa day
31 December	Maintain weight over Christmas	Keep up exercise Two detox days	Fit into new little black dress!

Bullet Guide: Ten Rules for Guaranteed Weight Loss

The bigger picture

You're in this for the long haul, so consider the **bigger picture** ... one biscuit is not a problem, a 'blowout' weekend won't undo everything, but you need to keep it all in **balance**.

Balancing your calorie intake does not have to be a constant **denial** of all the foods you want to eat. Follow a more balanced approach whereby you **offset indulgences** with extra exercise or lower calorie days, keeping your overall calorie intake in balance with energy expenditure.

This long-term **credit–debit arrangement** allows you to have your cake – and eat it!

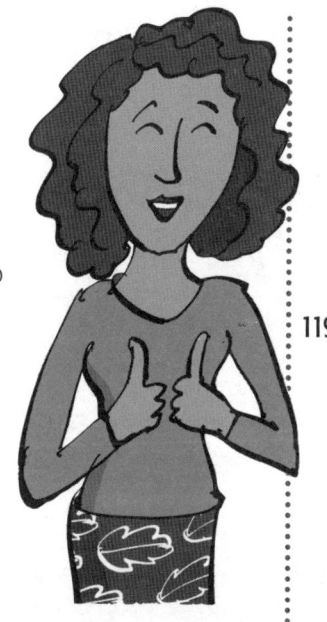

Further reading

Food Doctor Diet by Ian Marber (Dorling Kindersley, 2003).

Food for Health – The Essential Guide by Sara Kirkham (Need2Know, 2010).

Get into Running by Sara Kirkham (Hodder Headline, 2010).

GI: How to Succeed Using a Glycaemic Index Diet (HarperCollins, 2005).

How to Cook the Weight Watchers Way by Becky Johnson and Joy Skipper (Simon and Schuster, 2005).

Lose Weight, Gain Energy, Get Healthy by Sara Kirkham (Hodder Headline, 2010).

Weight Loss – The Essential Guide by Sara Kirkham (Need2Know, 2010).